HISTOLOGICAL TYPING OF GASTRIC AND OESOPHAGEAL TUMOURS

INTERNATIONAL HISTOLOGICAL CLASSIFICATION OF TUMOURS

No. 18

HISTOLOGICAL TYPING OF GASTRIC AND OESOPHAGEAL TUMOURS

K. OOTA

Head, WHO International Reference Centre for the Histological Classification of Gastro-oesophageal Tumours, Faculty of Medicine, University of Tokyo, Japan

in collaboration with

L. H. SOBIN

Pathologist, World Health Organization
Geneva, Switzerland

and pathologists in thirteen countries

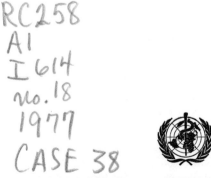

WORLD HEALTH ORGANIZATION

GENEVA

1977

ISBN 92 4 176018 4

PRINTED IN SWITZERLAND

LIST OF PARTICIPANTS

WHO International Reference Centre for the Histological Classification of Gastro-oesophageal Tumours, * Faculty of Medicine, University of Tokyo, Tokyo, Japan **

Head of Centre

Dr K. OOTA (1970–1976) **
Dr T. IMAI (1968–1970) ***

Consultant Pathologists

Dr I. KINO, Department of Pathology, University of Hamamatsu School of Medicine, Hamamatsu, Japan

Dr T. NAGAYO, Department of Pathology, Aichi Cancer Centre, Nagoya City, Japan

Participants

Dr O. BJARNASON, Department of Pathology, University of Iceland, Reykjavik, Iceland

Dr O. JÄRVI, Department of Pathological Anatomy, University of Turku, Finland

Dr N. I. KOLYCHEVA, Oncological and Radiological Research Institute, Alma Ata, Kazakhstan, USSR

Dr J. MICHALANY, Department of Pathology, Escola Paulista de Medicina, São Paulo, Brazil

Dr B. C. MORSON, Research Department, St Mark's Hospital, London, England

Dr N. M. SMIRNOV, Laboratory of Pathology, Research Institute of Oncology, Leningrad, USSR

Dr L. H. SOBIN, Cancer, World Health Organization, Geneva, Switzerland

---

* Following a decision taken by the World Health Organization in 1974 in the interest of uniformity, all WHO-designated centres have been renamed WHO Collaborating Centres; thus the above centre is now known as the WHO Collaborating Centre for the Histological Classification of Gastro-oesophageal Tumours.

** Present address: Tokyo Metropolitan Institute of Gerontology, Sakaecho, Itabishiku, Tokyo, Japan.

*** Cancer Research Institute, Faculty of Medicine, Kyushu University, Fukuoka, Japan.

Dr D. A. WOOD, Cancer Research Institute, University of California, Medical Center, San Francisco, CA, USA

Dr A. WYNN-WILLIAMS, Department of Laboratory Medicine, Hamilton General Hospital, Hamilton, Ontario, Canada

Reviewers

Dr P. CORREA, National Cancer Institute, National Institutes of Health, Bethesda, MD, USA

Dr K. ELSTER, Pathology Institute, Municipal Hospital, Bayreuth, Federal Republic of Germany

Dr L. R. FINLAY-JONES, Department of Pathology, Royal Perth Hospital, Perth, Australia

Dr R. LOUBIÈRE, Department of Pathology, Faculty of Medicine, Abidjan, Ivory Coast

Dr M. RAPAPORT, Hospital Fernandez, Buenos Aires, Argentina

Dr R. VANĚČEK, Second Department of Pathology, Charles University, Prague, Czechoslovakia

CONTENTS

Colour photomicrographs

The photomicrographs reproduced in this volume were taken by Mrs O. Frey, Cinégram S.A., Geneva, Switzerland.

GENERAL PREFACE TO THE SERIES

Among the prerequisites for comparative studies of cancer are international agreement on histological criteria for the classification of cancer types and a standardized nomenclature. At present, pathologists use different terms for the same pathological entity, and furthermore the same term is sometimes applied to lesions of different types. An internationally agreed classification of tumours, acceptable alike to physicians, surgeons, radiologists, pathologists and statisticians, would enable cancer workers in all parts of the world to compare their findings and would facilitate collaboration among them.

In a report published in 1952,[1] a subcommittee of the WHO Expert Committee on Health Statistics discussed the general principles that should govern the statistical classification of tumours and agreed that, to ensure the necessary flexibility and ease in coding, three separate classifications were needed according to (1) anatomical site, (2) histological type, and (3) degree of malignancy. A classification according to anatomical site is available in the International Classification of Diseases.[2]

The question of establishing a universally accepted classification by histological type has received much attention during the last 20 years and a particularly valuable Atlas of Tumor Pathology—*already numbering more than 40 volumes—is being published in the USA by the Armed Forces Institute of Pathology under the auspices of the National Research Council. An* Illustrated Tumour Nomenclature *in English, French, German, Latin, Russian, and Spanish has also been published by the International Union Against Cancer (UICC).*

In 1956 the WHO Executive Board passed a resolution[3] requesting the Director-General to explore the possibility that WHO might organize centres in various parts of the world and arrange for the collection of human tissues and their histological classification. The main purpose of such centres would be to develop histological definitions of cancer types and to facilitate the wide adoption of a uniform nomenclature. This resolution was endorsed by the Tenth World Health Assembly in May 1957[4] and the following month a Study Group on Histological Classification of Cancer Types met in Oslo to

---

[1] *Wld Hlth Org. techn. Rep., Ser.*, 1952, No. 53, p. 45.
[2] World Health Organization (1967) *Manual of the International Statistical Classification of Diseases, Injuries, and Causes of Death*, 1965 revision, Geneva.
[3] *Off. Rec. Wld Hlth Org.*, 1956, **68**, 14 (Resolution EB17.R40).
[4] *Off. Rec. Wld Hlth Org.*, 1957, **79**, 467 (Resolution WHA10.18).

advise WHO on its implementation. The Group recommended criteria for selecting tumour sites for study and suggested a procedure for the drafting of histological classifications and testing their validity. Briefly, the procedure is as follows :

For each tumour site, a tentative histopathological typing and classification is drawn up by a group of experts, consisting of up to ten pathologists working in the field in question. An international reference centre and a number of collaborating laboratories are then designated by WHO to evaluate the proposed classification. These laboratories exchange histological preparations, accompanied by clinical information. The histological typing is then made in accordance with the proposed classification. Subsequently, one or more technical meetings are called by WHO to facilitate an exchange of opinions and the classification is amended to take account of criticisms.

In addition to preparing the publication and the photomicrographs for it, the reference centre produces up to 100 sets of microscope slides showing the major histological types for distribution to national societies of pathology.

Since 1958, WHO has established 23 centres covering tumours of the lung ; breast ; soft tissues ; oropharynx ; bone ; ovaries ; salivary glands ; thyroid ; skin ; male urogenital tract ; jaws ; female genital tract ; stomach and oesophagus ; intestines ; central nervous system ; liver, biliary tract and pancreas ; upper respiratory tract ; eye ; and endocrine glands ; as well as oral precancerous conditions ; the leukaemias and lymphomas ; comparative oncology ; and exfoliative cytology. This work has involved more than 300 pathologists from over 50 countries. A number of these centres have completed their work, and most of their classifications have already been published (see page 6).

The World Health Organization is indebted to the many pathologists who have participated and are participating in this large undertaking. The pioneer work of many other international and national organizations in the field of histological classification of tumours has greatly facilitated the task undertaken by WHO. Particular gratitude is expressed to the National Cancer Institute, USA, which, through the National Research Council and the USA National Committee for the International Council of Societies of Pathology, is providing financial support to accelerate this work. Finally, WHO wishes to record its appreciation of the valuable help it has received from the International Council of Societies of Pathology (ICSP) in proposing participants and in undertaking to distribute copies of the classifications, with corresponding sets of microscope slides, to national societies of pathology all over the world.

PREFACE TO
HISTOLOGICAL TYPING OF GASTRIC AND
OESOPHAGEAL TUMOURS

The WHO International Reference Centre for the Histological Classification of Gastro-oesophageal Tumours was established in 1968 at the Cancer Research Institute, Faculty of Medicine, Kyushu University, Fukuoka, Japan and was transferred to the Department of Pathology, Faculty of Medicine, University of Tokyo, Japan in 1970.

The Centre distributed histological sections from selected cases to the participants, who are listed on page 5, for typing according to a tentative classification drawn up at a WHO consultation in 1967. In all, about 200 cases were thus studied and were reviewed at meetings in 1972 and 1974 attended by the participants. The classification, its definitions, and its nomenclature were amended at these meetings in the light of this study. The classification and selected cases were reviewed by a second group of pathologists designated by WHO (see page 6). At the meeting in 1974 the present classification was adopted.

The colour photomicrographs appearing in this book are also available as a collection of transparencies intended especially for teaching purposes. To help those who might wish to know the corresponding terms in French, Russian, and Spanish, translations of the classification into these languages are also given, immediately following the English version.

It will, of course, be appreciated that the classification reflects the present state of knowledge and modifications are almost certain to be needed as experience accumulates. Although the present classification has been adopted by the members of the group, it necessarily represents a view from which some pathologists may wish to dissent. It is nevertheless hoped that in the interests of international cooperation, all pathologists will try to use the classification as put forward. Criticisms and suggestions for its improvement will be welcomed. These should be sent to the World Health Organization, 1211 Geneva 27, Switzerland.

The publications in the series International Histological Classification of Tumours *are not intended to serve as textbooks but rather to promote the adoption of a uniform terminology and categorization of tumours that will facilitate and improve communication among cancer workers. For this reason the literature references have intentionally been kept to a minimum and readers are referred to standard works on the subject for extensive bibliographies.*

INTRODUCTION

This classification is based primarily on the microscopic characteristics of the tumours and therefore is concerned with morphologically identifiable cell types and histological patterns as seen with conventional light microscopy.

Grading of certain types of malignant tumours by the use of a modifying phrase to indicate the degree of their differentiation is widely practised. Although it has been considered to be of prognostic significance in certain cases, it may be of doubtful value in others. It deserves continuing investigation in relation to all types. The general approach that has been adopted in this volume, particularly in respect of carcinomas, is to grade them into three categories in the following manner:

Well differentiated—a carcinoma with histological and cellular features that closely resemble normal epithelium of similar type.

Moderately differentiated—a carcinoma intermediate between well differentiated and poorly differentiated.

Poorly differentiated—a carcinoma with histological and cellular features that only barely resemble normal epithelium of similar type.

A malignant tumour may contain areas with different degrees of differentiation. Because it has been postulated that the biological behaviour of such a tumour will be a reflection of its most poorly differentiated component, it should be graded on this basis. Grading should not be made, however, at the growing edges of the tumour or at the portions directly adjacent to ulcerative or inflammatory processes.

It must be emphasized that factors other than the histological types and grades have important influences on the behaviour of tumours and prognosis. Special consideration should be given to the extent of tumour spread at the time of diagnosis. It is recommended that a statement as to the deepest anatomical layer of the wall, e.g., mucosal, submucosal, muscular, or serosal, reached by the tumour follow the typing and grading.

Among other microscopic features that might be related to tumour behaviour are vascular invasion, demarcation, cellular reaction, inflammatory infiltration, and desmoplasia.

Malignant tumours, especially carcinomas of the stomach, may contain areas with different histological types, as well as different degrees of differentiation. It is recommended that such tumours should be first categorized according to the predominant features (type and differentiation) and notes added indicating the presence of other histological types and degrees of differentiation. It should be recognized that in some cases it may be impossible to tell whether a variation in type has developed or whether a tumour is composed of two independent primary tumours, i.e., collision tumours. If different tumours are present in the same specimen a diagnosis should be given for each and they should be separately categorized.

Electron microscopy and histochemistry may be of great value in investigating the nature of certain tumours. However, in most instances diagnosis of oesophageal and gastric tumours can be made by means of conventional light microscopy with routine staining methods. In most cases haematoxylin-eosin staining is sufficient for diagnostic purposes. However, special stains may be necessary for further evaluation. The use of methods to identify mucins (neutral, acid, and sulfated) is of particular value in distinguishing varieties of gastric carcinomas.

Time-honoured terms have generally been retained in this publication. Synonyms are listed only if they have been widely used or if they are considered to be important for an understanding of the disease. In such cases, the preferred term is given first, followed by the synonym in brackets.

HISTOLOGICAL CLASSIFICATION
OF OESOPHAGEAL TUMOURS

I. EPITHELIAL TUMOURS

A. BENIGN
1. Squamous cell papilloma

B. MALIGNANT
1. Squamous cell carcinoma
2. Adenocarcinoma
3. Adenoid cystic carcinoma
4. Mucoepidermoid carcinoma
5. Adenosquamous carcinoma
6. Undifferentiated carcinoma

II. NON-EPITHELIAL TUMOURS

A. BENIGN
1. Leiomyoma
2. Others

B. MALIGNANT
1. Leiomyosarcoma
2. Others

III. MISCELLANEOUS TUMOURS

A. CARCINOSARCOMA

B. MALIGNANT MELANOMA

C. OTHERS

IV. SECONDARY TUMOURS

V. UNCLASSIFIED TUMOURS

VI. TUMOUR-LIKE LESIONS

A. HETEROTOPIAS

B. CONGENITAL CYSTS

C. FIBROVASCULAR POLYP [FIBROUS POLYP]

―――――

HISTOLOGICAL CLASSIFICATION
OF GASTRIC TUMOURS

I. EPITHELIAL TUMOURS

A. BENIGN

    1. Adenoma
      (*a*) papillary [villous]
      (*b*) tubular
      (*c*) papillotubular

B. MALIGNANT

    1. Adenocarcinoma [1]
      (*a*) papillary
      (*b*) tubular
      (*c*) mucinous
      (*d*) signet-ring cell carcinoma

    2. Adenosquamous carcinoma

    3. Squamous cell carcinoma

    4. Undifferentiated carcinoma

    5. Unclassified carcinoma

II. CARCINOID TUMOURS

III. NON-EPITHELIAL TUMOURS

A. SMOOTH MUSCLE TUMOURS

    1. Leiomyoma

    2. Leiomyoblastoma

    3. Leiomyosarcoma

B. OTHERS

---

[1] For the classification of carcinomas into " intestinal " and " diffuse " types, see page 41.

IV. HAEMATOPOIETIC AND LYMPHOID NEOPLASMS

A. LYMPHOSARCOMA

B. RETICULOSARCOMA

C. HODGKIN'S DISEASE

D. PLASMACYTOMA

E. OTHERS

V. MISCELLANEOUS TUMOURS

VI. SECONDARY TUMOURS

VII. UNCLASSIFIED TUMOURS

VIII. TUMOUR-LIKE LESIONS

A. HYPERPLASTIC POLYP

B. INFLAMMATORY FIBROID POLYP [EOSINOPHILIC GRANULOMATOUS POLYP]

C. LYMPHOID HYPERPLASIA

D. HETEROTOPIAS
1. Pancreatic heterotopia
2. Heterotopia of Brunner's glands
3. Submucosal heterotopia of gastric glands

E. HAMARTOMAS
1. Peutz-Jeghers polyp
2. Others

F. JUVENILE POLYP

G. GIANT RUGAL HYPERTROPHY

H. OTHERS

CLASSIFICATION HISTOLOGIQUE
DES TUMEURS ŒSOPHAGIENNES

I. TUMEURS ÉPITHÉLIALES

A. BÉNIGNES
   1. Papillome épidermoïde

B. MALIGNES
   1. Carcinome * épidermoïde
   2. Adénocarcinome
   3. Carcinome adénoïde kystique [cylindrome]
   4. Carcinome mucoépidermoïde
   5. Carcinome adénosquameux
   6. Carcinome indifférencié

II. TUMEURS NON ÉPITHÉLIALES

A. BÉNIGNES
   1. Léiomyome
   2. Autres

B. MALIGNES
   1. Léiomyosarcome
   2. Autres

III. TUMEURS DIVERSES

A. CARCINOSARCOME

B. MÉLANOME MALIN

C. AUTRES

---

* Carcinome et adénocarcinome sont synonymes d'épithélioma et d'épithélioma glandulaire.

IV. TUMEURS SECONDAIRES

V. TUMEURS NON CLASSÉES

VI. LÉSIONS PSEUDOTUMORALES

A. HÉTÉROTOPIES

B. KYSTES CONGÉNITAUX

C. POLYPE FIBROVASCULAIRE [POLYPE FIBREUX]

CLASSIFICATION HISTOLOGIQUE
DES TUMEURS GASTRIQUES

I. TUMEURS ÉPITHÉLIALES

A. BÉNIGNES

1. Adénome
   (a) papillaire [villeux]
   (b) tubulaire
   (c) tubulo-papillaire

B. MALIGNES

1. Adénocarcinome [1]
   (a) papillaire
   (b) tubulaire
   (c) mucineux
   (d) carcinome à cellules en bague à chaton [carcinome à cellules indépendantes mucipares]

2. Carcinome adénosquameux

3. Carcinome épidermoïde

4. Carcinome indifférencié

5. Carcinome non classé

II. TUMEURS CARCINOÏDES

III. TUMEURS NON ÉPITHÉLIALES

A. TUMEURS DES MUSCLES LISSES

1. Léiomyome

2. Léiomyoblastome

3. Léiomyosarcome

B. AUTRES

---

[1] Pour la classification des carcinomes de type « intestinal » et « diffus », voir page 41.

IV. TUMEURS HÉMATOPOIÉTIQUES ET LYMPHOÏDES

A. LYMPHOSARCOME

B. RÉTICULOSARCOME

C. MALADIE DE HODGKIN

D. PLASMOCYTOME

E. AUTRES

V. TUMEURS DIVERSES

VI. TUMEURS SECONDAIRES

VII. TUMEURS NON CLASSÉES

VIII. LÉSIONS PSEUDOTUMORALES

A. POLYPE HYPERPLASIQUE

B. POLYPE FIBREUX INFLAMMATOIRE [POLYPE GRANULOMATEUX ÉOSINO-PHILE]

C. HYPERPLASIE LYMPHOÏDE

D. HÉTÉROTOPIES
   1. Hétérotopie pancréatique
   2. Hétérotopie des glandes de Brunner
   3. Hétérotopie sous-muqueuse des glandes gastriques

E. HAMARTOMES
   1. Polype de Peutz-Jeghers
   2. Autres

F. POLYPE JUVÉNILE

G. GASTROPATHIE À PLIS GÉANTS

H. AUTRES.

ГИСТОЛОГИЧЕСКАЯ КЛАССИФИКАЦИЯ ОПУХОЛЕЙ ПИЩЕВОДА

I. ЭПИТЕЛИАЛЬНЫЕ ОПУХОЛИ

A. Доброкачественные

    1. Плоскоклеточная папиллома

B. Злокачественные

    1. Плоскоклеточный рак

    2. Аденокарцинома

    3. Железисто–кистозный рак

    4. Мукоэпидермоидный рак

    5. Железисто–плоскоклеточный рак

    6. Недифференцированный рак

II. НЕЭПИТЕЛИАЛЬНЫЕ ОПУХОЛИ

A. Доброкачественные

    1. Лейомиома

    2. Другие

B. Злокачественные

    1. Лейомиосаркома

    2. Другие

III. СМЕШАННЫЕ ОПУХОЛИ

A. Карциносаркома

B. Злокачественная меланома

C. Другие

IV. ВТОРИЧНЫЕ ОПУХОЛИ

V. НЕКЛАССИФИЦИРУЕМЫЕ ОПУХОЛИ

VI. ОПУХОЛЕПОДОБНЫЕ ПОРАЖЕНИЯ

A. Гетеротопии

B. Врожденные кисты

C. Фиброваскулярный полип [фиброзный полип]

ГИСТОЛОГИЧЕСКАЯ КЛАССИФИКАЦИЯ
ОПУХОЛЕЙ ЖЕЛУДКА

I. ЭПИТЕЛИАЛЬНЫЕ ОПУХОЛИ

А. Доброкачественные

    1. Аденома
        а) папиллярная [ворсинчатая]
        б) тубулярная
        в) папиллотубулярная

Б. Злокачественные

    1. Аденокарцинома[1]
        а) папиллярная
        б) тубулярная
        в) муцинозная
        г) перстневидноклеточный рак

    2. Железисто–плоскоклеточный рак

    3. Плоскоклеточный рак

    4. Недифференцированный рак

    5. Неклассифицируемый рак

II. КАРЦИНОИДНЫЕ ОПУХОЛИ

III. НЕЭПИТЕЛИАЛЬНЫЕ ОПУХОЛИ

А. Опухоли гладких мышц

    1. Лейомиома

    2. Лейомиобластома

    3. Лейомиосаркома

Б. Другие

---

[1] Для классификации на типы «кишечный» и «диффузный» смотри страницу 41.

IV. ГЕМАТОПОЭТИЧЕСКИЕ И ЛИМФОИДНЫЕ ОПУХОЛИ

А. Лимфосаркома

Б. Ретикулосаркома

В. Болезнь Ходжкина

Г. Плазмоцитома

Д. Другие

V. СМЕШАННЫЕ ОПУХОЛИ

VI. ВТОРИЧНЫЕ ОПУХОЛИ

VII. НЕКЛАССИФИЦИРУЕМЫЕ ОПУХОЛИ

VIII. ОПУХОЛЕПОДОБНЫЕ ПОРАЖЕНИЯ

А. Гиперпластический полип

Б. Воспалительный фиброзный полип [эозинофильный
грануломатозный полип]

В. Лимфоидная гиперплазия

Г. Гетеротопии
   1. Гетеротопия ткани поджелудочной железы
   2. Гетеротопия бруннеровых желез
   3. Гетеротопия желудочных желез в подслизистом слое

Д. Гамартомы
   1. Полип Пейтца–Егерса
   2. Другие

Е. Ювенильный полип

Ж. Гигантские гипертрофированные складки

З. Другие

CLASIFICACION HISTOLOGICA DE LOS TUMORES ESOFAGICOS

I. TUMORES EPITELIALES

A. BENIGNOS
   1. Papiloma espinocelular

B. MALIGNOS
   1. Carcinoma espinocelular
   2. Adenocarcinoma
   3. Carcinoma adenoide cístico
   4. Carcinoma mucoepidermoide
   5. Carcinoma adenoescamoso
   6. Carcinoma indiferenciado

II. TUMORES NO EPITELIALES

A. BENIGNOS
   1. Leiomioma
   2. Otros

B. MALIGNOS
   1. Leiomiosarcoma
   2. Otros

III. TUMORES MISCELÁNEOS

A. CARCINOSARCOMA

B. MELANOMA MALIGNO

C. OTROS

IV. TUMORES SECUNDARIOS

V. TUMORES NO CLASIFICADOS

VI. LESIONES SEUDOTUMORALES

A. HETEROTOPIAS

B. QUISTES CONGÉNITOS

C. PÓLIPO FIBROVASCULAR [PÓLIPO FIBROSO]

———————

CLASIFICACION HISTOLOGICA DE LOS TUMORES GASTRICOS

I. TUMORES EPITELIALES

A. Benignos

   1. Adenoma
     a) papilar [velloso]
     b) tubular
     c) tubulopapilar

B. Malignos

   1. Adenocarcinoma [1]
     a) papilar
     b) tubular
     c) mucinoso
     d) carcinoma de células en anillo de sello

   2. Carcinoma adenoescamoso

   3. Carcinoma espinocelular

   4. Carcinoma indiferenciado

   5. Carcinoma no clasificado

II. TUMORES CARCINOIDES

III. TUMORES NO EPITELIALES

A. Tumores de músculo liso

   1. Leiomioma

   2. Leiomioblastoma

   3. Leiomiosarcoma

B. Otros

---

[1] Para la clasificación de carcinomas en tipos « intestinal » y « difuso », ver pág. 41.

IV. NEOPLASIAS DEL TEJIDO LINFOIDE Y HEMATOPOYÉTICO

A. LINFOSARCOMA

B. RETICULOSARCOMA

C. ENFERMEDAD DE HODGKIN

D. PLASMOCITOMA

E. OTROS

V. TUMORES MISCELÁNEOS

VI. TUMORES SECUNDARIOS

VII. TUMORES NO CLASIFICADOS

VIII. LESIONES SEUDOTUMORALES

A. PÓLIPO HIPERPLÁSICO

B. PÓLIPO FIBROIDE INFLAMATORIO [PÓLIPO GRANULOMATOSO EOSINOFÍLICO]

C. HIPERPLASIA LINFOIDE

D. HETEROTOPIAS
    1. Heterotopia pancreática
    2. Heterotopia de las glándulas de Brunner
    3. Heterotopia submucosa de glándulas gástricas

E. HAMARTOMAS
    1. Pólipo de Peutz-Jeghers
    2. Otros

F. PÓLIPO JUVENIL

G. GASTROPATÍA DE PLIEGUES GIGANTES

H. OTROS

DEFINITIONS AND EXPLANATORY NOTES

OESOPHAGEAL TUMOURS

I. EPITHELIAL TUMOURS

A. BENIGN

1. *Squamous cell papilloma* (Fig. 1–2): A benign tumour composed of squamous cells covering finger-like processes with cores derived from the lamina propria. It is very rare.

There is an extremely rare inherited condition of multiple papillomas of the oesophagus in association with hyperkeratosis of the palms and soles. Oesophageal carcinoma frequently occurs in the affected individuals.[1] Multiple papillomas of the oesophagus have also been found in patients with acanthosis nigricans.

B. MALIGNANT

1. *Squamous cell carcinoma* (Fig. 3–15): A malignant epithelial tumour composed of cells resembling those of squamous epithelium.

This is by far the most common malignant tumour of the oesophagus. It is usually graded as well, moderately, or poorly differentiated. Well-differentiated tumours are those with abundant amounts of keratin, easily demonstrated intercellular bridges, and minimal nuclear and cellular pleomorphism. Poorly differentiated tumours are those with no or virtually no keratin and intercellular bridges or with marked cellular and nuclear pleomorphism. Moderately differentiated tumours are those intermediate between well and poorly differentiated.

In some poorly differentiated tumours, the cells are spindle-shaped and may be mistaken for sarcoma. This variant of squamous cell carcinoma is called *spindle-cell carcinoma* (Fig. 6).

An uncommon form of squamous cell carcinoma consisting of squamous cell nests and spindle cell stroma has been referred to as pseudosarcoma

---

[1] Howel-Evans, W. et al. *Quarterly Journal of Medicine* (N.S.), 27, 413-429 (1958).

(Fig. 7–10). The proportions of the two components can vary in different cases. It is often polypoid and shows areas of *in situ* squamous cell carcinoma in the overlying and adjacent epithelium.

Verrucous carcinoma is a variant of squamous cell carcinoma that has been rarely reported in the oesophagus. It is a papillary growth of high differentiation (Fig. 11–12).

After radiotherapy squamous cell carcinomas of the oesophagus usually show extensive changes in their histological appearances. Loss or loosening of cell cohesion with degenerative atypia may be seen as an early response. The tumour cells can also disappear almost completely, leaving fibrotic areas in which small groups of bizarre eosinophilic cell bodies containing pyknotic or fragmented nuclei are embedded. Foreign body granulomas may be seen around the keratinized material. Groups of tumour cells in the regrowth phase may appear undifferentiated.

In situ squamous cell carcinoma is a lesion with cytological features of carcinoma but with no invasion of the basement membrane (Fig. 14–15). It should be distinguished from various degrees of *dysplasia*, i.e., epithelial atypia in a flat mucosa, which occur in the oesophagus and should be recorded according to conventional criteria, e.g., mild, moderate, or severe (Fig. 16).

2. *Adenocarcinoma* (Fig. 17–18): A malignant tumour of glandular type epithelium. It may have a papillary pattern.

Primary adenocarcinoma can arise from heterotopic gastric mucosa in the oesophagus or from submucosal mucous glands. Adenocarcinomas with small foci of squamous metaplasia (adenoacanthoma) should be classified under adenocarcinoma.

It may be difficult or impossible to tell whether an adenocarcinoma found in the lower end of the oesophagus is the result of spread from a tumour in the stomach or is a true primary growth of the oesophagus.

3. *Adenoid cystic carcinoma* (Fig. 19): A malignant epithelial tumour having a characteristic cribriform structure. The tumour cells are of two types: cells similar to those lining the normal mucous gland ducts and cells of myoepithelial type. The cells form small duct-like structures or larger masses dispersed around cystic spaces, as in similar tumours of the salivary glands. The tumour is rare in the oesophagus.

The term cylindroma has been used for this neoplasm.

4. *Mucoepidermoid carcinoma* (Fig. 20): A tumour characterized by the presence of an intimate mixture of squamous cells, mucus-secreting cells, and cells of intermediate type.

The relative proportions of the three cell types vary. The squamous cell component is usually present in the form of clumps or multi-layered masses beneath the mucus-secreting epithelium. Keratinization is uncommon. These tumours are identical to the mucoepidermoid tumours of salivary glands. They are rare in the oesophagus.

5. *Adenosquamous carcinoma* : A tumour in which adenocarcinomatous and squamous carcinomatous components are intermingled.

It should be distinguished from foci of squamous metaplasia in an adenocarcinoma (adenoacanthoma).

6. *Undifferentiated carcinoma* (Fig. 21–22): A malignant epithelial tumour that shows no glandular or squamous structure.

A distinct but rare form of undifferentiated carcinoma referred to as *oat-cell carcinoma* has been described in the oesophagus. It resembles that seen in the lung and has been associated with hormone production by the tumour.

II. NON-EPITHELIAL TUMOURS

These are classified according to the WHO scheme published elsewhere.[1]

A. BENIGN

1. *Leiomyoma*

This is the most common type of benign non-epithelial tumour encountered in the oesophagus.

2. *Others*

B. MALIGNANT

1. *Leiomyosarcoma*

This is the most frequently encountered malignant non-epithelial tumour in the oesophagus.

2. *Others*

III. MISCELLANEOUS TUMOURS

A. CARCINOSARCOMA: A tumour consisting of an intimate mixture of carcinoma and sarcoma growing together as a single tumour.

---

[1] Enzinger, F. M., Lattes, R. & Torloni, H. *Histological typing of soft tissue tumours*, Geneva, World Health Organization, 1969 (*International Histological Classification of Tumours*, No. 3).

True carcinosarcoma has been described on very rare occasions. It may be extremely difficult to differentiate this type of tumour from " pseudosarcoma " (see page 33) unless the mesenchymal origin of the sarcomatous parts is indicated by specific differentiation, e.g., cartilage, either in the primary growth or in the metastatic foci. The carcinomatous parts are usually squamous.

B. Malignant melanoma (Fig. 23–24)

Malignant melanoma in the oesophagus is much more commonly metastatic than primary. Junctional activity is an important feature of primary tumours, but may be obscured in advanced tumours.

C. Others

Carcinoid tumours and choriocarcinoma have on rare occasions been described as arising in the oesophagus.

IV. SECONDARY TUMOURS

V. UNCLASSIFIED TUMOURS

Primary benign or malignant tumours that cannot be placed in any of the categories described above.

VI. TUMOUR-LIKE LESIONS

A. Heterotopias (Fig. 25)

Small islands of gastric heterotopic tissue are found in the upper oesophagus. In the lower oesophagus, the heterotopic tissue is often more extensive and usually continuous with that of the stomach. Gastric heterotopia in the lower oesophagus is either congenital or is associated with chronic oesophagitis.

Intestinal metaplasia can occur in these heterotopias.

B. Congenital cysts

These malformations are either lined entirely by epithelium that is ciliated, squamous, or gastric or by more than one of these.

C. Fibrovascular polyp [fibrous polyp] (Fig. 26): A polyp composed of a core of fibrous or adipose connective tissue and blood vessels covered by thickened but otherwise normal squamous epithelium.

GASTRIC TUMOURS

I. EPITHELIAL TUMOURS

A. BENIGN

1. *Adenoma* (Fig. 27–34): A benign tumour of glandular epithelium having varying degrees of cellular atypia and showing papillary and/or tubular structures.

   (a) *Papillary* [*villous*] : An adenoma composed of pointed or blunt finger-like processes with cores derived from the lamina propria.

   (b) *Tubular:* An adenoma composed predominantly of branching tubules embedded in or surrounded by lamina propria.

In flat, tubular adenomas, the abnormal epithelium can occupy the upper portion of the mucosa while the subjacent part of the mucosa may remain unchanged or show cystic dilatation of glands. Mucus secretion is diminished in tubular adenomas. This has also been called adenomatous polyp.

Gastric adenomas seen in cases of adenomatosis (familial polyposis) of the colon are usually of tubular type and are flat rather than polypoid.

   (c) *Papillotubular:* An adenoma that has both papillary and tubular patterns or a pattern that appears to be intermediate between papillary and tubular.

This has been known as tubulovillous or villoglandular adenoma.

Gastric adenomas are more often slightly elevated lesions with a flat surface rather than having a stalk. Whereas adenomas with prominent stalks are common in the large intestine, they are uncommon in the stomach and must be differentiated from hyperplastic polyp. Although several adenomas may occur in a stomach, when numerous polyps are found these are usually hyperplastic (see p. 44).

Adenomas of the stomach are also characterized by cellular type as follows: those composed entirely of intestinal epithelium; those composed entirely of superficial gastric, i.e., foveolar, epithelium; and those composed of a mixture of these epithelial cells. Dysplastic changes may be encountered in any of these cellular types. Mitotic figures are often increased and are uniformly distributed (see the discussion of carcinoma in situ, p. 40).

B. MALIGNANT

1. *Adenocarcinoma :* A malignant tumour of glandular epithelium that contains tubular, acinar, or papillary structures.

Most carcinomas of the stomach are adenocarcinomas. The tumour cells sometimes resemble normal gastric epithelium and sometimes intestinal epithelium, particularly in their surface structure and secretory activities. Cells of the Paneth type may be present in variable numbers. In addition, cells with argentaffin or argyrophilic granules may be scattered in an adenocarcinoma, but they are usually few in number and do not alter the classification.

Variation in the histological appearances in different parts of an adenocarcinoma is often very striking. For example, an adenocarcinoma sometimes exhibits different histological features depending upon the layer in which the tumour grows. A papillary adenocarcinoma in the mucosa may appear as a mucinous adenocarcinoma in the deeper layers. In the diagnosis of gastric adenocarcinoma, it is recommended that the typing be based on predominance with mention of minor components in the description.

(a) *Papillary adenocarcinoma* (Fig. 35–36): An adenocarcinoma composed of pointed or blunt finger-like epithelial processes with fibrous cores.

The tumour cells are cylindrical or cuboidal and usually maintain well-polarized surface orientation but they can also show moderate to severe cellular and nuclear pleomorphism. Although this subtype may show some tubular formation the papillary pattern is evident, particularly in cystic structures.

Papillary adenocarcinoma typically grows as a polypoid mass into the gastric lumen; when deep invasion occurs peripheral demarcation is sharp and infiltration with leucocytes is common.

(b) *Tubular adenocarcinoma* (Fig. 37–44): An adenocarcinoma composed predominantly of branching tubules embedded in or surrounded by fibrous stroma.

The size of the cross-sections of the tubules varies and there can be cystic dilatation. The tumour cells are cylindrical or cuboidal but may be flattened by accumulation of mucin in the dilated lumens. Adenocarcinomas with acinar structures are included in this category.

(c) *Mucinous adenocarcinoma* (Fig. 45–46): An adenocarcinoma in which substantial amounts of mucin are retained within the tumour and which is usually visible to the naked eye.

In some varieties of this tumour, the distended glands are filled with mucin, which may escape into the interstitium; in other varieties disintegrated epithelial components appear as chains or groups of cells floating in lakes of mucin. In such cases limited numbers of signet-ring cells may be seen. In some tumours the cytological elements may be obscured by the mucin content, but nevertheless an attempt should be made to assess the degree of differentiation.

The term mucinous adenocarcinoma is used synonymously with mucoid, mucous, colloid, and muconodular adenocarcinoma.

(d) Signet-ring cell carcinoma (Fig. 47–50): An adenocarcinoma with a predominant component of isolated tumour cells containing prominent amounts of mucin.

Three types of tumour cells have been described in this carcinoma: (*i*) a cell with an intracytoplasmic cyst filled with acid mucin, giving the classical signet-ring appearance; (*ii*) a tumour cell with eosinophilic cytoplasmic granules containing neutral mucin with a slightly eccentric nucleus; and (*iii*) a tumour cell whose cytoplasm is distended with secretory granules of acid mucin appearing like a goblet cell. These three cell types may occur independently or in combination within any one tumour.

This tumour tends to infiltrate diffusely and is often associated with considerable fibrosis (" scirrhous "). So-called " linitis plastica " often corresponds to this type of tumour, involving the entire stomach.

Extensive fibrosis may obscure the nature of a signet-ring cell carcinoma. Stains for mucin may clarify this problem. The presence of lipid-laden macrophages in the lamina propria must be differentiated from intramucosal signet-ring cell carcinoma.

Signet-ring cell carcinoma is synonymous with mucocellular carcinoma.

* *
*

Adenocarcinoma of the stomach may be graded in the following manner:

Well differentiated—an adenocarcinoma with a glandular and cellular structure that in most cases closely resembles metaplastic intestinal epithelium.

Moderately differentiated—an adenocarcinoma intermediate between well differentiated and poorly differentiated.

Poorly differentiated—an adenocarcinoma that has a glandular and cellular structure which can be recognized only with difficulty.

* *
*

Certain terms, defined as follows, are used to describe growth patterns of gastric carcinomas:

" *Solid* "—the cells are closely packed and the tumours have a well-defined boundary; they are usually undifferentiated but may contain acinar structures.

" *Scirrhous* "—the tumour cells are few relative to the fibrous stroma; this pattern is characteristic of so-called " linitis plastica " but may not be reproduced in metastatic deposits;

" *Intramucosal* "—infiltration of tumour in the lamina propria and confined to the mucous membrane (above the muscularis mucosae). This term is *not* synonymous with carcinoma in situ. Intramucosal carcinoma of the stomach can metastasize to regional lymph nodes. Focal adenocarcinoma and signet-ring cell carcinoma in polypoid lesions of the stomach should be considered forms of intramucosal carcinoma.

" *Superficial spreading carcinoma* "—extensive lateral spread of the tumour, primarily in the mucosa and superficial submucosa. It is *not* synonymous with intramucosal carcinoma.

Carcinoma in situ, in the stomach, is an expression applied by some to mucosal lesions including adenomas, in which the epithelial cells show conspicuous changes described as severe atypia or dysplasia. The term should not be used if there is invasion of cells across the basement membrane of the glands (see intramucosal carcinoma, above).

2. *Adenosquamous carcinoma* (Fig. 51): A single tumour in which both adenocarcinomatous and squamous carcinomatous elements are present. This condition is distinct from small foci of squamous metaplasia, which may occur in gastric adenocarcinoma (adeno-acanthoma), and from collision tumours.

3. *Squamous cell carcinoma* (Fig. 52): A malignant epithelial tumour composed of cells resembling those of squamous epithelium.

In the majority of cases reported as gastric squamous cell carcinoma, small foci of adenocarcinoma have been found. Most squamous cell carcinomas of the cardia are the result of spread from a tumour in the oesophagus.

4. *Undifferentiated carcinoma* (Fig. 53–54): A malignant epithelial tumour that has no glandular structure or other features to indicate definite differentiation.

Terms such as carcinoma simplex, medullary carcinoma, and trabecular carcinoma have been used by different authors for these tumours, but their use is not recommended.

5. *Unclassified carcinoma:* A malignant epithelial tumour that cannot be placed in any of the categories described above.

* *
*

Classification into intestinal and diffuse types

In addition to the traditional classification given above, gastric carcinomas may also be subdivided into intestinal and diffuse types.[1] This distinction can have importance both for epidemiological and clinical studies.

The *intestinal type* is typically characterized by a predominance of glandular epithelium composed of elements resembling intestinal columnar cells with more or less distinct brush borders and in many cases also goblet cells. As with intestinal metaplasia the columnar cells show mucus secretion. The cells of intestinal type cancer may also show clear cell differentiation. In the cases of intestinal type carcinomas, intestinal metaplastic mucosa is often widely spread in the vicinity of the neoplasm. The neoplasm is mostly well demarcated. Fig. 35–39 and 45 are examples of the intestinal type.

The *diffuse type* of carcinoma may show, particularly in the surface or superficial part of the tumour, some glandular arrangements but is mainly characterized by poorly cohesive, rather small rounded cells, with wide and diffuse infiltration of the gastric wall. Many of the cells contain mucus and can show the typical signet-ring shape but non-secreting cells also occur. The type of mucus does not differ from that of intestinal type carcinomas. The neoplasm is poorly demarcated. Fig. 46, 48, and 49 are examples of the diffuse type.

Paneth cells and argentaffin cells as well as interstitial mucus may be present in both intestinal and diffuse types.

	Intestinal	Diffuse
Tubules	Well developed	Poorly developed
Mucus	Present	Present
Pattern	Well-demarcated margin	Poorly demarcated margin
	Compact	Dispersed

Whereas the majority of gastric carcinomas can be subdivided into intestinal and diffuse types, a minority cannot be so classified. These include tumours with about equal proportions of intestinal and diffuse characteristics and others that are undifferentiated and have a solid growth pattern. These are placed in an *indeterminate* category (Fig. 44). Squamous cell carcinoma and adenosquamous carcinoma are separately categorized.

---

[1] According to Laurén (Laurén, P. *Acta pathol. microbiol. scand.*, **64**: 31, 1965), based on histogenetic studies by Järvi and Laurén (Järvi, O. & Laurén, P. *Acta pathol. microbiol. scand.*, **29**: 26 (1951).

II. CARCINOID TUMOURS (Fig. 55–56)

Carcinoid tumours are rare in the stomach. They are usually non-argentaffin but may be argyrophil and usually behave in a malignant manner.

Carcinoid tumours arise from the basal part of the gastric mucosa, and are found much more frequently in the antrum than in the corpus. They tend to infiltrate the submucosa early, often appearing as a submucosal tumour. The overlying mucosa may be elevated or ulcerated. Typically the carcinoid tumour is composed of uniform cells of small to medium size with poorly defined cell boundaries. They have round regular nuclei and are arranged in sheets, cords, and clusters. Attempts to form rosettes and acinar structures are sometimes noted. On electron microscopy the cytoplasm contains characteristic granules. These granules may appear argentaffin [1] (e.g., by the Fontana method), argyrophil [2] (e.g., by the Bodian method), or non-reactive. Some carcinoid tumours consist of columnar cells that form tubular lumens reminiscent of adenocarcinoma. They show infiltrative borders and appear to behave in a more aggressive manner, like adenocarcinomas.

III. NON-EPITHELIAL TUMOURS

These are, in general, classified and defined according to the WHO scheme published elsewhere.[3] Only those most commonly encountered in the stomach are listed here.

A. SMOOTH MUSCLE TUMOURS

1. *Leiomyoma* (Fig. 59)

This is the most common non-epithelial tumour of the stomach. Typical histological features are interlacing bundles of uniform eosinophilic spindle-shaped cells surrounded by reticulin fibres and containing elongated nuclei with blunt ends. Mitotic figures are absent or sparse. Leiomyomas may become calcified. Commonly they are small and can be multiple. They may be intramural or protrude from the outer or inner surface of the stomach. Ulceration is common in large growths. Tumours with prominent nuclear palisading and hyaline change must not be mistaken for neurilemmomas.

---

[1] *Argentaffin*: silver-positive with a technique that does not use an external reducing agent.

[2] *Argyrophil*: silver-positive with a technique that uses an external reducing agent.

[3] Enzinger, F. M., Lattes, R. & Torloni, H. *Histological typing of soft tissue tumours*, Geneva, World Health Organization, 1969 (*International Histological Classification of Tumours*, No. 3).

2. *Leiomyoblastoma* (Fig. 60)

This is a distinctive tumour also known as epithelioid leiomyoma. It is characterized by predominantly rounded or polygonal cells with a clear space partially or completely surrounding the nucleus. The clear space is considered to be an artefact and may not appear in well-fixed specimens. Mitotic figures are scanty or absent. Myofibrils cannot usually be demonstrated but transitions towards typical elongated smooth muscle cells are seen occasionally. The tumour, which sometimes reaches an enormous size, usually arises from the muscle coat of the stomach wall of adult patients. Its behaviour is very difficult to predict. The majority of leiomyoblastomas follow a benign clinical course despite the presence of pleomorphism; some, however, are known to have metastasized.

3. *Leiomyosarcoma* (Fig. 61–62)

This is the most common malignant soft tissue tumour of the stomach. It is often ulcerated and consequently cystic and its morphology is frequently altered by these changes. Central necrosis may lead to fistula formation.

The differential diagnosis of leiomyosarcoma from highly cellular leiomyomas may be impossible. The most important single criterion for malignancy is the presence of mitotic figures, especially abnormal ones.

B. Others

Neurilemmoma, neurogenic sarcoma (malignant schwannoma), granular cell tumour (myoblastoma), lipoma, glomus tumour, haemangioma, haemangiopericytoma, and lymphangioma can occur in the stomach.

IV. HAEMATOPOIETIC AND LYMPHOID NEOPLASMS (Fig. 63–64)

Lymphosarcoma and reticulosarcoma are the commonest primary lymphomas of the stomach, while Hodgkin's disease is rare. The distinction between reticulosarcomas and undifferentiated carcinomas may be difficult. Ulceration and consequent inflammation can modify the histological appearance of gastric lymphomas but diagnosis can be facilitated by examining regional lymph nodes. Plasmacytoma has been rarely described as arising in the stomach. Lymphomas must be distinguished from lymphoid hyperplasia (see p. 45).

V. MISCELLANEOUS TUMOURS

The very rare occurrence of primary choriocarcinoma (Fig. 57–58), teratoma, carcinosarcoma, and malignant melanoma of the stomach has been described. Foci of adenocarcinoma may be present in a primary gastric choriocarcinoma.

VI. SECONDARY TUMOURS

VII. UNCLASSIFIED TUMOURS

Primary benign or malignant tumours that cannot be placed in any of the categories described above.

VIII. TUMOUR-LIKE LESIONS

A. HYPERPLASTIC POLYP (Fig. 67–68): A benign sessile or pedunculated polyp composed of irregular hyperplastic glands. The epithelium is mostly of the foveolar (i.e., superficial gastric) type, but pyloric (antral) glands, chief cells, and parietal cells may be present. Cellular atypia is usually absent but when present it is mild and focal.

Cystic change and superficial ulceration are common. Intestinal metaplasia is infrequent and usually focal. The stroma may contain bands of fibromuscular tissue and shows a variable amount of inflammatory cell infiltration.

Hyperplastic polyps can be single or multiple and are usually located in the antrum rather than the body of the stomach. When multiple, they are often distributed along the boundary of the antral and fundic mucosa. They are common lesions and must be differentiated from the much less frequent adenoma and Peutz-Jeghers polyp.

Hyperplastic polyp has also been called hyperplastic adenomatous polyp, inflammatory polyp, regenerative polyp, and gastritis polyposa.

B. INFLAMMATORY FIBROID POLYP [EOSINOPHILIC GRANULOMATOUS POLYP] (Fig. 69–70): A circumscribed lesion in a polypoid form composed of a background of fibroblasts, histiocytes and blood vessels, infiltrated by a variable number of, but sometimes numerous, eosinophil leukocytes. The blood vessels are typically surrounded by fibroblasts arranged in an onion-skin pattern.

Usually this lesion is well demarcated and found mainly in the submucosa and involves the basal portion of the mucosa and parts of the muscularis. Subsequent ulceration often occurs in the overlying mucosa.

This lesion is unrelated to histiocytosis X, eosinophilic gastritis, and the foreign body granulomatous reaction associated with certain parasites and food material.

C. Lymphoid hyperplasia (Fig. 65–66): A lesion in which there is a reactive type of lymphoid hyperplasia.

The lesion may be diffuse or localized and can be polypoid with infiltration by a mixture of lymphocytes, histiocytes, and plasma cells in the mucosa and submucosa. Lymphoid follicles with germinal centres are typically present. There may be associated ulceration and fibrosis. Absence of atypia of the lymphoid cells and presence of well-defined follicles indicate the benign reactive nature of the lesion.

D. Heterotopias

1. *Pancreatic heterotopia* (Fig. 71)

This is the most common variety of heterotopia. When smooth muscle and ducts are the only components the lesion has been known as " adenomyoma " or " myoepithelial hamartoma ".

2. *Heterotopia of Brunner's glands*

This is characterized by compact glands in the submucosa, typically partitioned by bands of smooth muscle.

3. *Submucosal heterotopia of gastric glands* (Fig. 72)

This consists of gastric glandular elements of any type located in the submucosa. These may show dilatation.

E. Hamartomas

1. *Peutz-Jeghers polyp* (Fig. 73–74): A lesion composed of an excess of essentially normal glands with cores of branching bands of smooth muscle, derived from the muscularis mucosae.

The glands may show hyperplasia and cystic change but there is no cellular atypia. It is more commonly multiple as part of the syndrome of gastro-intestinal polyposis.[1]

2. *Others*

F. Juvenile polyp: A lesion composed of tubules and cysts lined by normal foveolar epithelium, separated from one another by an excess of lamina propria.

These lesions can be complicated by ulceration and secondary infection leading to reactive hyperplasia of the epithelium. It is usually

---

[1] See: Morson, B. C. & Sobin, L, H. *Histological typing of intestinal tumours*, Geneva, World Health Organization, 1976 (*International Histological Classification of Tumours*, No. 15).

multiple as part of the syndrome of juvenile polyposis of the gastro-intestinal tract [1].

G. GIANT RUGAL HYPERTROPHY (Fig. 75–76): Diffuse rugal hypertrophy, predominantly of the fundus and body of the stomach, with hyperplasia of any or all of the glandular components. It is usually diffuse but may be localized.

This lesion is also known as hyperplastic gastropathy and has been included under the title of Menetrier's disease.

The term giant hypertrophic gastritis should be avoided.

H. OTHERS

This category includes parasitic granulomas (Fig. 77), e.g., due to anisakis, and chronic peptic ulcer with abundant fibrous tissue.

Irregularly thickened foci of gastric mucosa with tubules and mucus-filled cysts lined by foveolar epithelium are found in the Cronkhite-Canada syndrome [2] (Fig. 78).

---

[1] See: Morson, B. C. & Sobin, L. H. *Histological typing of intestinal tumours*, Geneva, World Health Organization, 1976 (*International Histological Classification of Tumours*, No. 15).

[2] Cronkhite, L. W. & Canada, W. J. *New Engl. J. Med.*, 252: 1011(1955).

INDEX

Unless otherwise stated, all the preparations shown in the photomicrographs reproduced on the following pages were stained with haematoxylin-eosin.

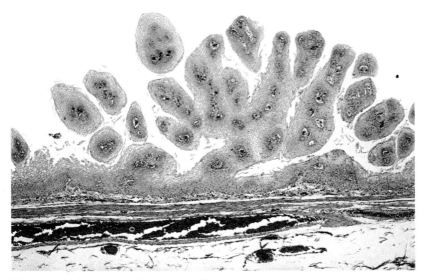

Fig. 1. Squamous cell papilloma, oesophagus

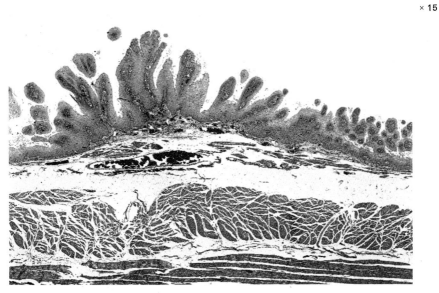

Fig. 2. Squamous cell papillomas, oesophagus
From a patient with acanthosis nigricans. The entire oesophagus contained small papillomas

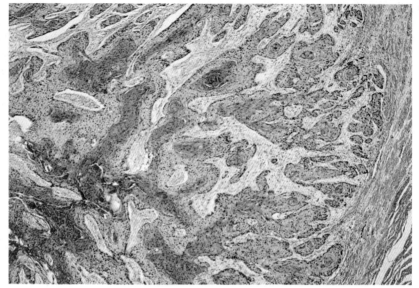

Fig. 3. Squamous cell carcinoma, oesophagus
Well differentiated

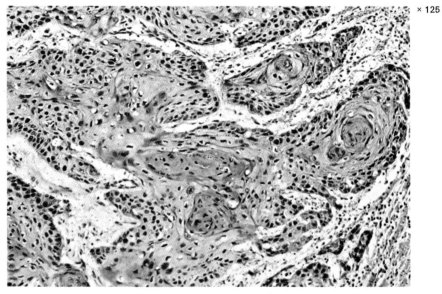

Fig. 4. Squamous cell carcinoma, oesophagus
Well differentiated. Same case as Fig. 3

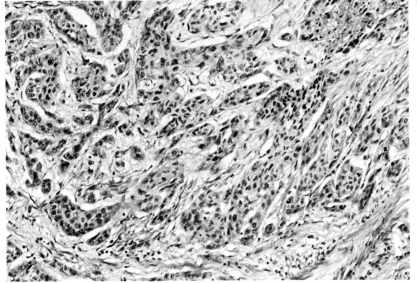

× 145

Fig. 5. Squamous cell carcinoma, oesophagus
Moderately differentiated

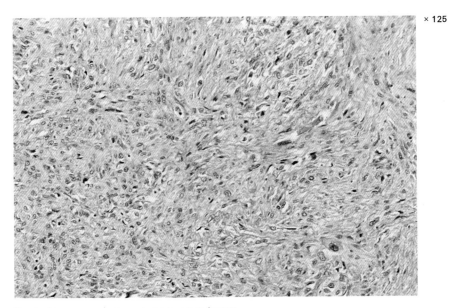

× 125

Fig. 6. Squamous cell carcinoma, oesophagus
Poorly differentiated. Spindle cell variant

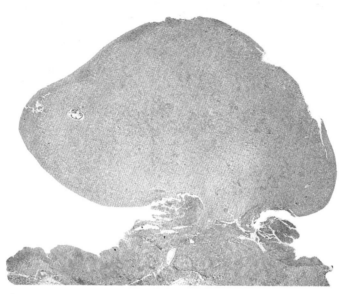

Fig. 7. Squamous cell carcinoma, oesophagus
Typical polypoid appearance of so-called pseudosarcoma

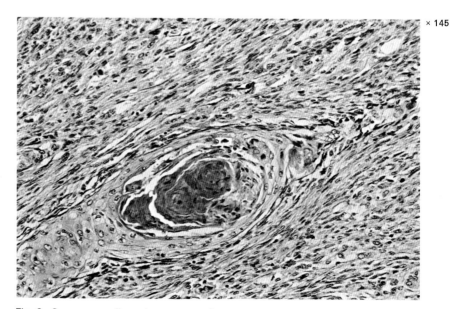

Fig. 8. Squamous cell carcinoma, oesophagus
Squamous cell nest with keratin in spindle cell stroma. So-called pseudosarcoma. Fig. 8–10
are from the same case

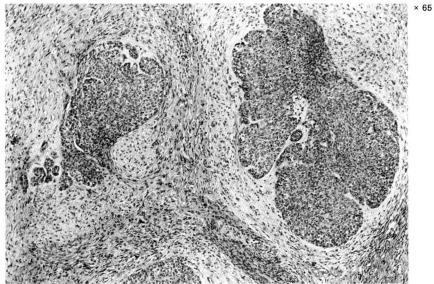

× 65

Fig. 9. Squamous cell carcinoma, oesophagus
Islands of squamous cells in sarcoma-like stroma

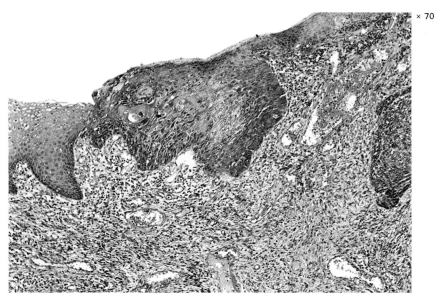

× 70

Fig. 10. Squamous cell carcinoma, oesophagus
Intraepithelial extension of tumour

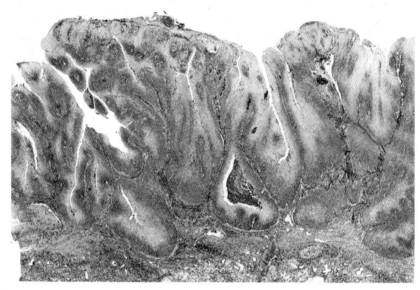

Fig. 11. Squamous cell carcinoma, oesophagus
Verrucous carcinoma

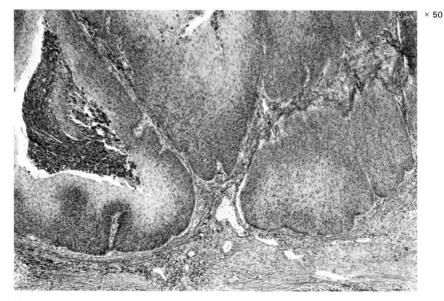

Fig. 12. Squamous cell carcinoma, oesophagus
Verrucous carcinoma. Typical blunt contours of deep margin

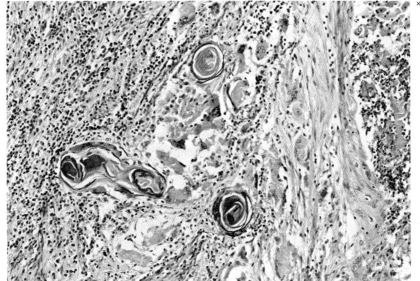

× 125

Fig. 13. Squamous cell carcinoma, oesophagus
Post-radiotherapy. Foreign body reaction with giant cells around keratin

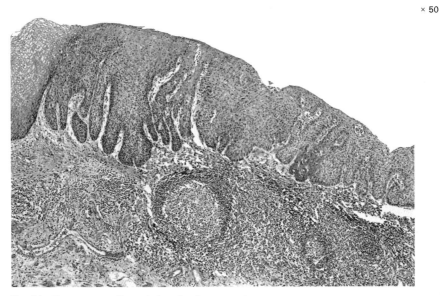

× 50

Fig. 14. Squamous cell carcinoma in situ, oesophagus
Well differentiated cells

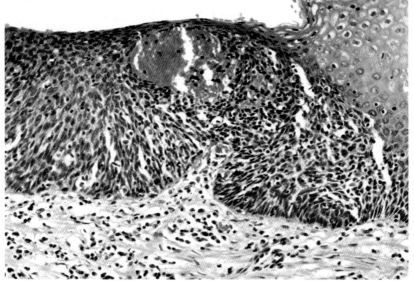

Fig. 15. Squamous cell carcinoma in situ, oesophagus
Poorly differentiated cells

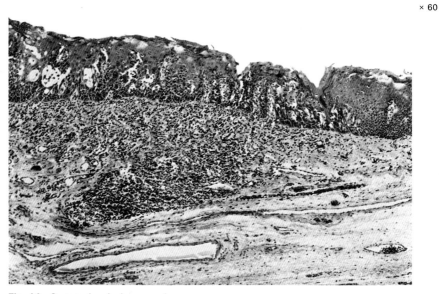

Fig. 16. Severe dysplasia, oesophagus
From a case of Plummer-Vinson syndrome

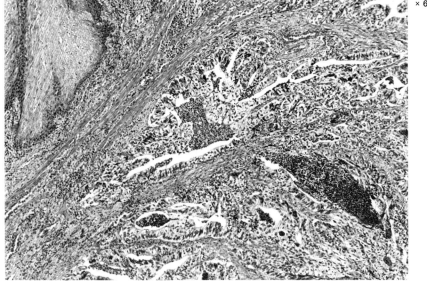

× 60

Fig. 17. Adenocarcinoma, oesophagus
Well differentiated. Necrotic material fills glandular lumens

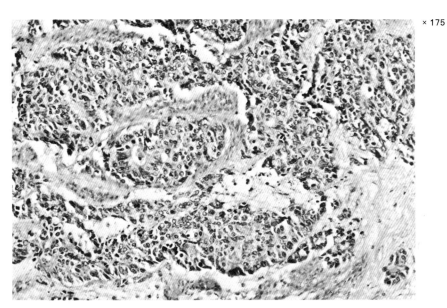

× 175

Fig. 18. Adenocarcinoma, oesophagus
Poorly differentiated

× 140

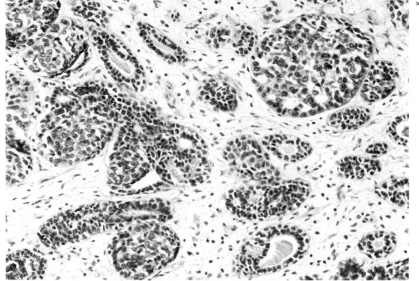

Fig. 19. Adenoid cystic carcinoma, oesophagus

× 50

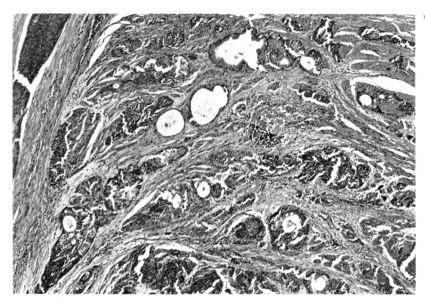

Fig. 20. Mucoepidermoid carcinoma, oesophagus

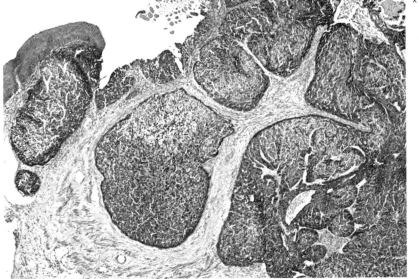

× 40

Fig. 21. Undifferentiated carcinoma, oesophagus

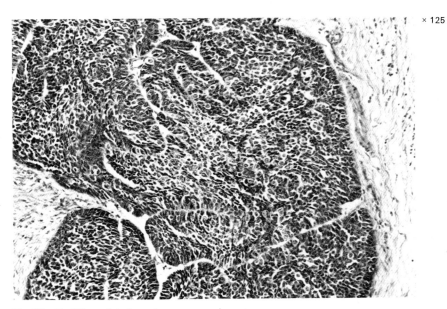

× 125

Fig. 22. Undifferentiated carcinoma, oesophagus

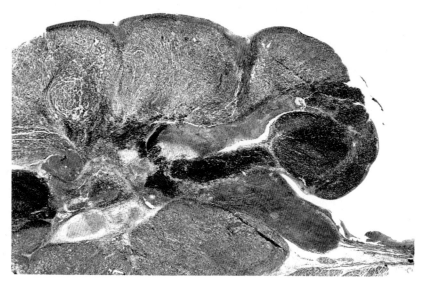

Fig. 23. Malignant melanoma, oesophagus
Heavily pigmented primary tumour

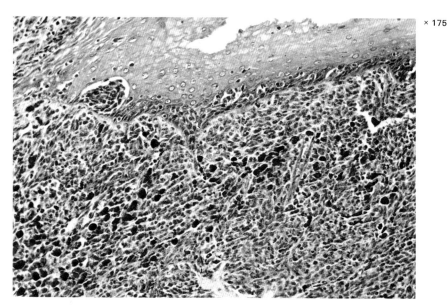

Fig. 24. Malignant melanoma, oesophagus
Same case as Fig. 23

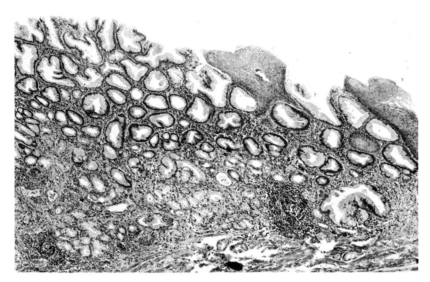

Fig. 25. Gastric heterotopia, upper oesophagus

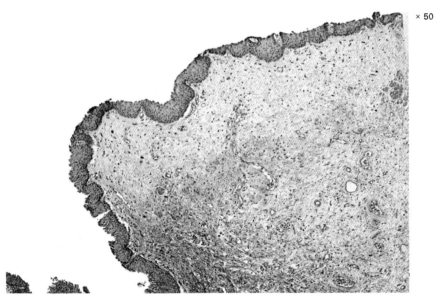

Fig. 26. Fibrovascular polyp, oesophagus

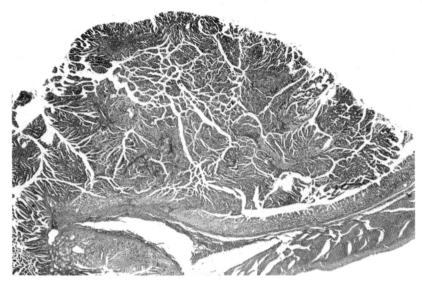

Fig. 27. Papillary adenoma, stomach

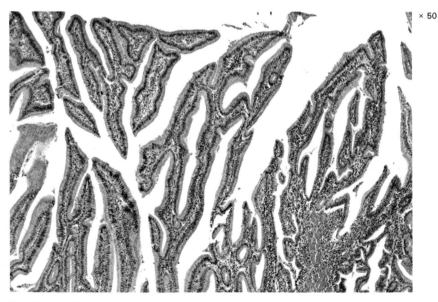

Fig. 28. Papillary adenoma, stomach
Same case as Fig. 27

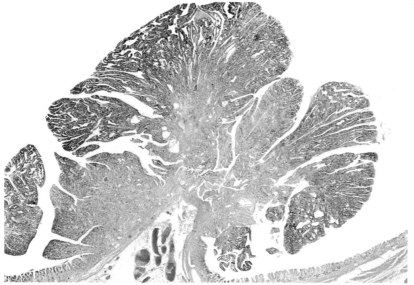

× 6

Fig. 29. Papillotubular adenoma, stomach

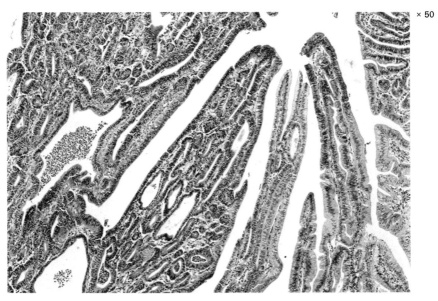

× 50

Fig. 30. Papillotubular adenoma, stomach
Same case as Fig. 29

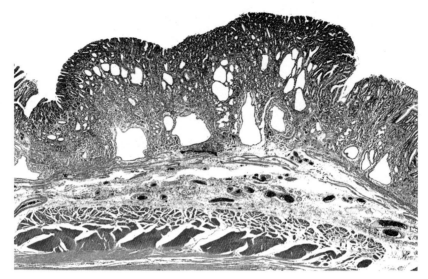

Fig. 31. Tubular adenoma, stomach
Flat rather than polypoid lesion

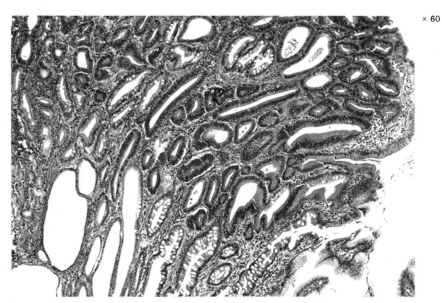

Fig. 32. Tubular adenoma, stomach
Same case as Fig. 31

× 9

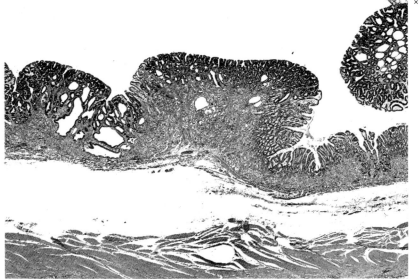

Fig. 33. Tubular adenomas, stomach
From a patient with familial polyposis of the colon

× 50

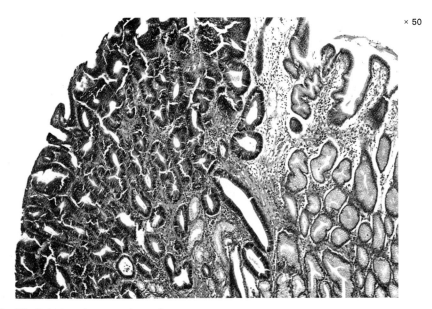

Fig. 34. Tubular adenoma, stomach
Same case as Fig. 33

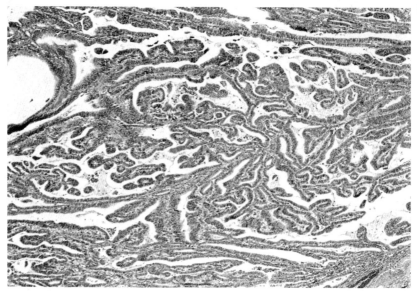

Fig. 35. Papillary adenocarcinoma, stomach
Well differentiated

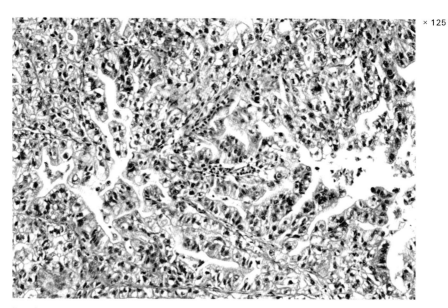

Fig. 36. Papillary adenocarcinoma, stomach
Moderately differentiated

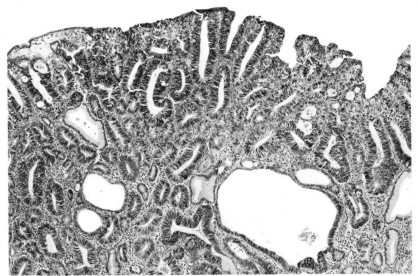

Fig. 37. Tubular adenocarcinoma, stomach
Well differentiated

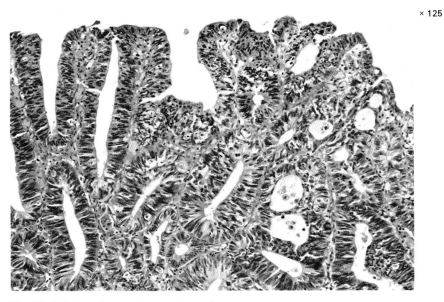

Fig. 38. Tubular adenocarcinoma, stomach
Well differentiated. Same case as Fig. 37

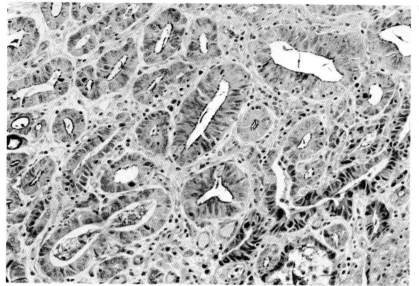

Fig. 39. Tubular adenocarcinoma, stomach
Well differentiated. Distinct brush borders. Alcian blue-PAS

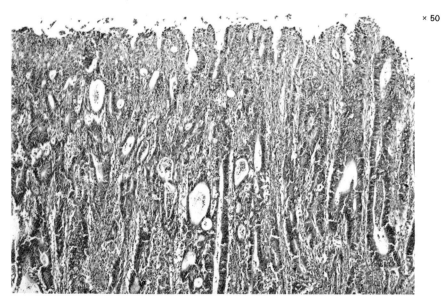

Fig. 40. Tubular adenocarcinoma, stomach
Moderately differentiated. Intramucosal infiltration

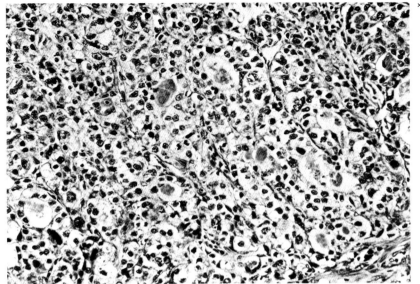

×190

Fig. 41. Tubular adenocarcinoma, stomach
Moderately differentiated

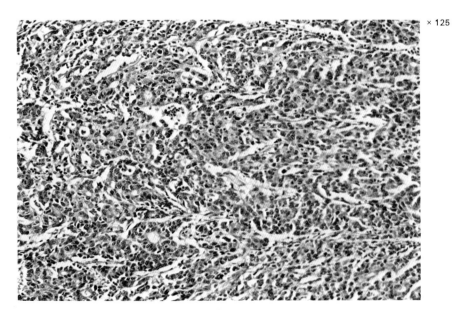

×125

Fig. 42. Tubular adenocarcinoma, stomach
Poorly differentiated

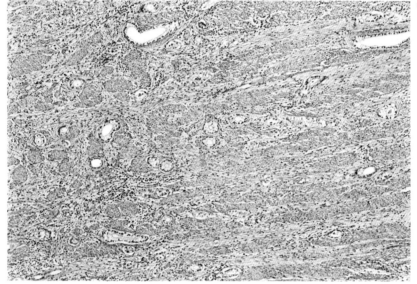

× 50

Fig. 43. Tubular adenocarcinoma, stomach
Scirrhous growth pattern

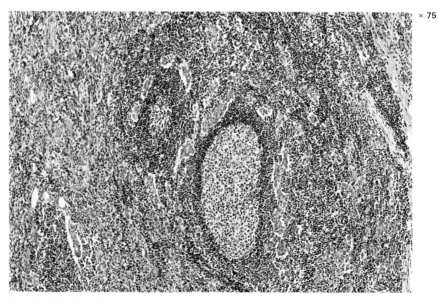

× 75

Fig. 44. Tubular adenocarcinoma, stomach
Poorly differentiated. Prominent lymphoid reaction

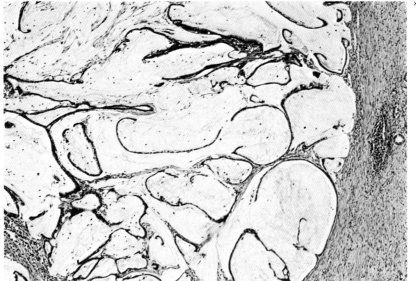

Fig. 45. Mucinous adenocarcinoma, stomach
Well differentiated

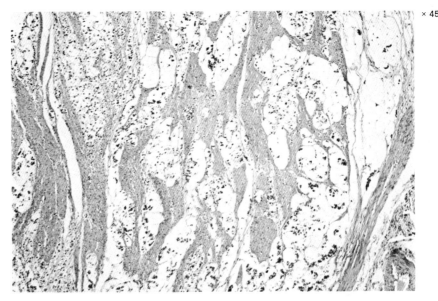

Fig. 46. Mucinous adenocarcinoma, stomach
Poorly differentiated

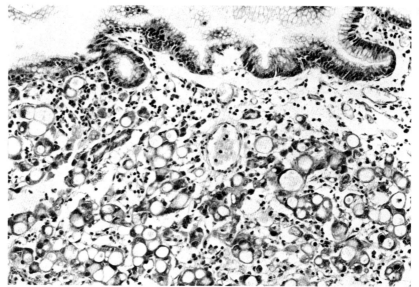

× 175

Fig. 47. Signet-ring cell carcinoma, stomach
Tumour cells with classic signet-ring appearance

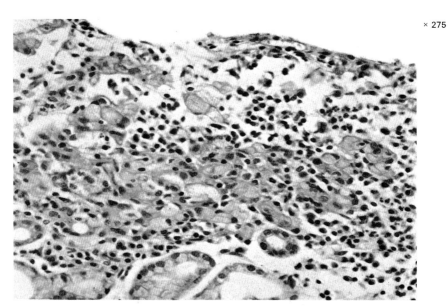

× 275

Fig. 48. Signet-ring cell carcinoma, stomach
Tumour cells with eosinophilic cytoplasmic granules

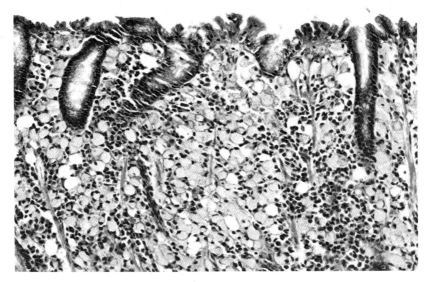

Fig. 49. Signet-ring cell carcinoma, stomach
Tumour cells with cytoplasm like that of goblet cells

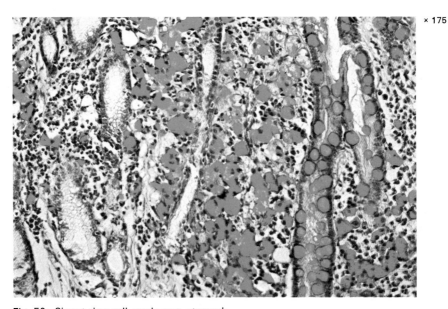

Fig. 50. Signet-ring cell carcinoma, stomach
Tumour cells with cytoplasm like that of goblet cells. Alcian blue

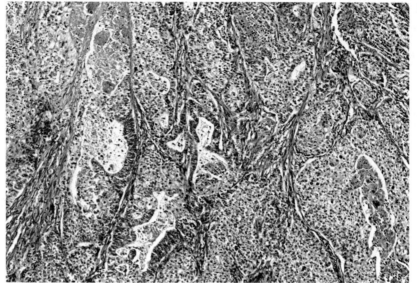

Fig. 51. Adenosquamous carcinoma, stomach

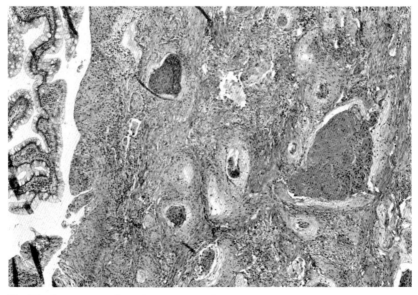

Fig. 52. Squamous cell carcinoma, stomach
Tumour located in antrum

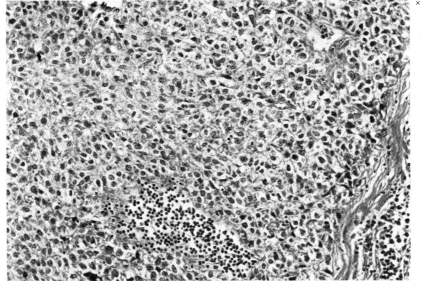

× 185

Fig. 53. Undifferentiated carcinoma, stomach
Solid growth pattern

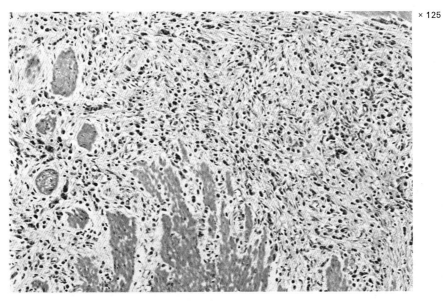

× 125

Fig. 54. Undifferentiated carcinoma, stomach
Scirrhous growth pattern

× 125

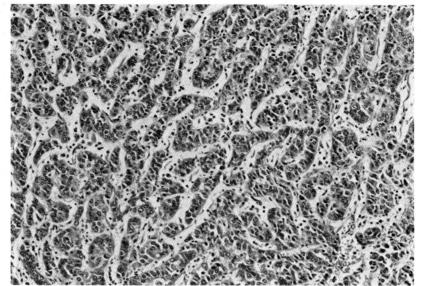

Fig. 55. Carcinoid tumour, stomach

× 125

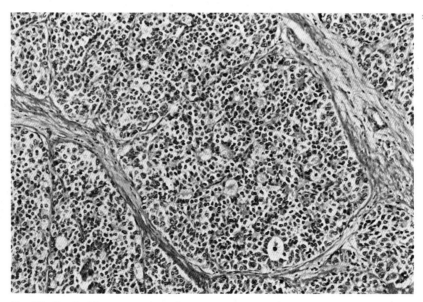

Fig. 56. Carcinoid tumour, stomach

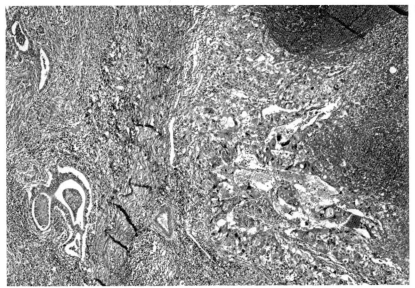

× 40

Fig. 57. Choriocarcinoma, stomach
Adenocarcinomatous foci in left portion of field. Adult male with high levels of chorionic gonadotropin

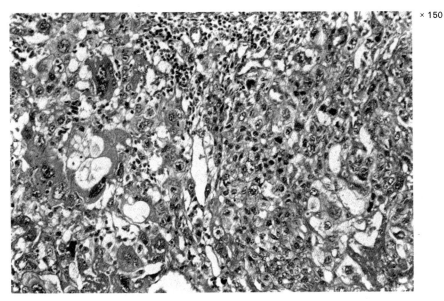

× 150

Fig. 58. Choriocarcinoma, stomach
Same case as Fig. 57

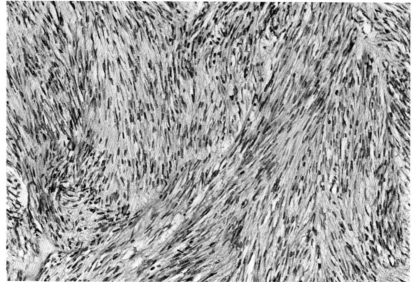

×130

Fig. 59. Leiomyoma, stomach

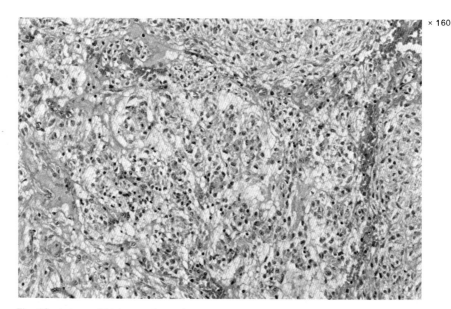

×160

Fig. 60. Leiomyoblastoma, stomach

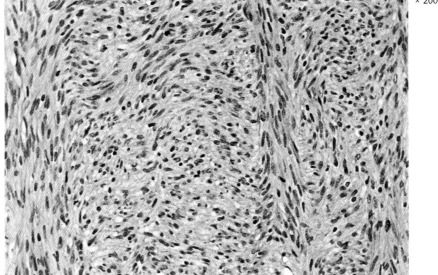

Fig. 61. Leiomyosarcoma, stomach
Well differentiated

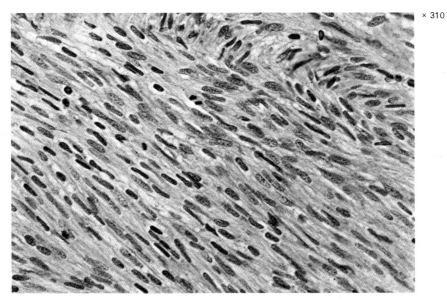

Fig. 62. Leiomyosarcoma, stomach
Mitoses. Same case as Fig. 61

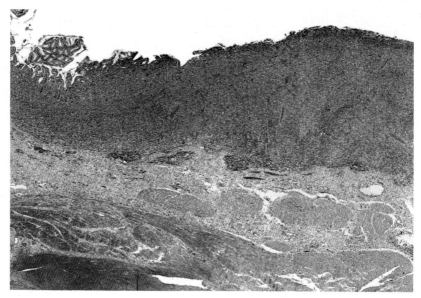

× 12

Fig. 63. Reticulosarcoma, stomach
Primary in stomach

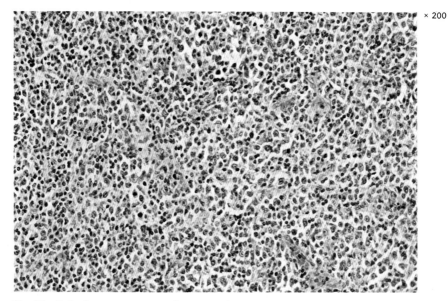

× 200

Fig. 64. Reticulosarcoma, stomach
Same case as Fig. 63

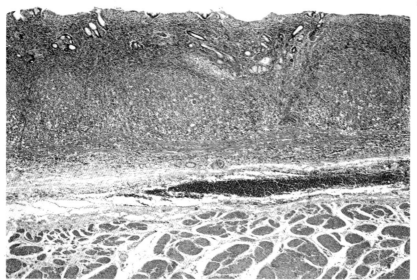

× 30

Fig. 65. Lymphoid hyperplasia, stomach
Germinal centres present

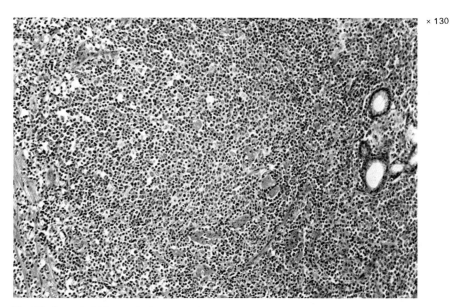

× 130

Fig. 66. Lymphoid hyperplasia, stomach
Same case as Fig. 65

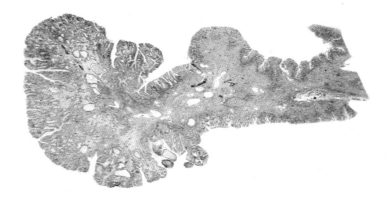

Fig. 67. Hyperplastic polyp, stomach

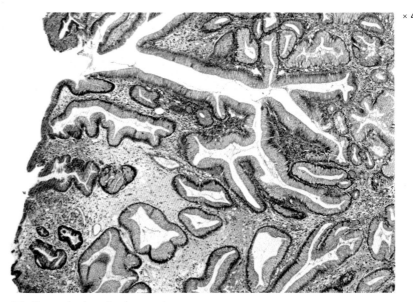

Fig. 68. Hyperplastic polyp, stomach

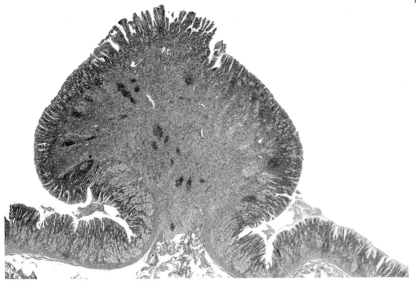

Fig. 69. Inflammatory fibroid polyp, stomach

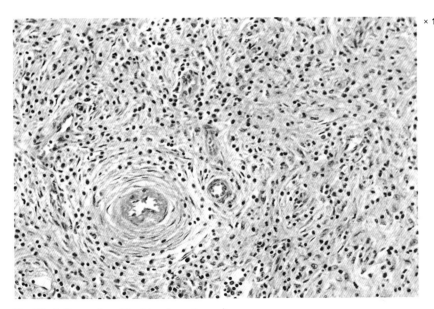

Fig. 70. Inflammatory fibroid polyp, stomach
Numerous eosinophil leucocytes. Typical perivascular onion-skin pattern of fibroblasts

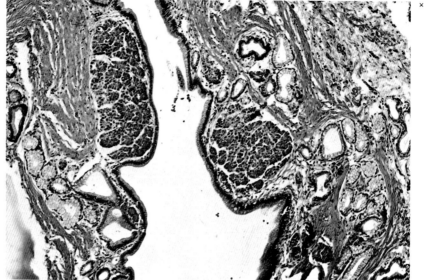

× 80

Fig. 71. Pancreatic heterotopia, stomach
Acinar and duct components present

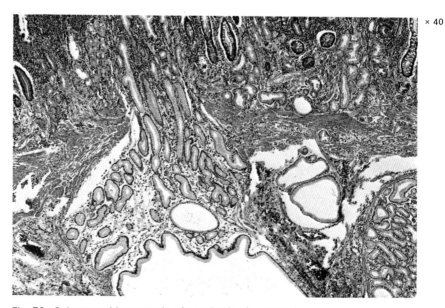

× 40

Fig. 72. Submucosal heterotopia of gastric glands, stomach
Muscularis mucosae separated by foveolar type glands. Glandular dilatation in deep portion

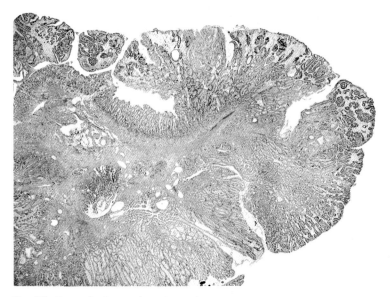

×7

Fig. 73. Peutz-Jeghers polyp, stomach

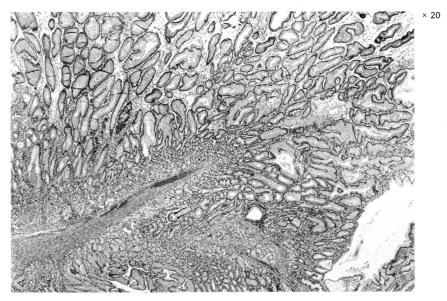

×20

Fig. 74. Peutz-Jeghers polyp, stomach
Same case as Fig. 73

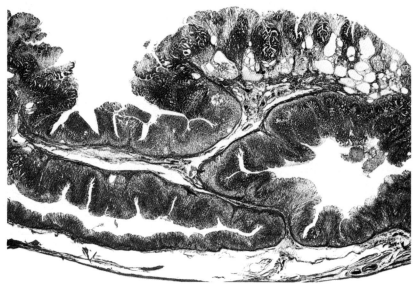

Fig. 75. Giant rugal hypertrophy, stomach

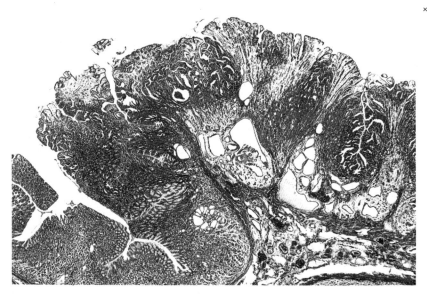

Fig. 76. Giant rugal hypertrophy, stomach
Same case as Fig. 75

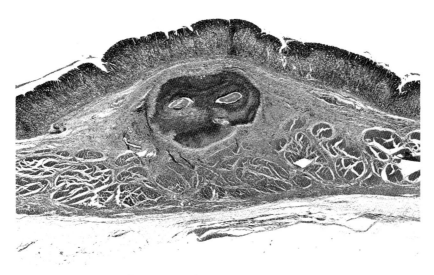

Fig. 77. Parasitic granuloma, stomach
Etiologic agent not identified

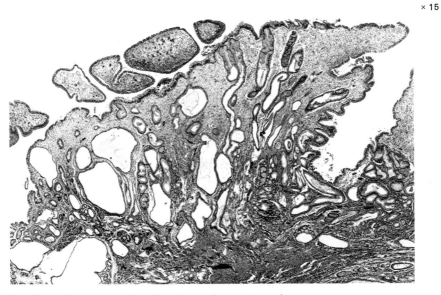

Fig. 78. Lesion of Cronkhite-Canada syndrome, stomach
Tubules and mucus-filled cysts lined by foveolar epithelium